GOUT DIET COOKBOOK

by Danielle Smith

© Copyright 2021 by Danielle Smith - All rights reserved.

The following Book is reproduced below with the goal of providing information that is as accurate and reliable as possible. Regardless, purchasing this Book can be seen as consent to the fact that both the publisher and the author of this book are in no way experts on the topics discussed within and that any recommendations or suggestions that are made herein are for entertainment purposes only. Professionals should be consulted as needed prior to undertaking any of the actions endorsed herein.
This declaration is deemed fair and valid by both the American Bar Association and the Committee of Publishers Association and is legally binding throughout the United States.
Furthermore, the transmission, duplication, or reproduction of any of the following work including specific information will be considered an illegal act irrespective of if it is done electronically or in print. This extends to creating a secondary or tertiary copy of the work or a recorded copy and is only allowed with the express written consent from the Publisher. All additional rights reserved.
The information in the following pages is broadly considered a truthful and accurate account of facts and as such, any inattention, use, or misuse of the information in question by the reader will render any resulting actions solely under their purview. There are no scenarios in which the publisher or the original author of this work can be in any fashion deemed liable for any hardship or damages that may befall them after undertaking the information described herein.
Additionally, the information in the following pages is intended only for informational purposes and should thus be thought of as universal. As befitting its nature, it is presented without assurance regarding its prolonged validity or interim quality. Trademarks that are mentioned are done without written consent and can in no way be considered an endorsement from the trademark holder.

table of content

- 7   WHAT IS A GOUT DIET
- 7   THE CAUSES OF GOUT
- 8   SIGNS AND SYMPTOMS
- 8   LIST OF FOOD TO AVOID AND RECOMMENDED FOOD
- 11   HOMEMADE REMEDIES FOR RELIEVING PAIN
- 14   PURINE TABLE INFORMATION
- 17   RECIPE FOR VEGETABLE BROTH
- 18   VEGETABLE AND SALADS RECIPES
- 45   SOUPS RECIPES
- 58   DESSERTS RECIPES
- 74   POTATOES AND VEGETABLE RECIPES

table of content

Spicy plantains	20
Spicy banana bread	21
Poppyseed salad	22
Seaweed salad	23
Bread salad	24
Spring salad	25
Papaya salad	26
Strawberry dressing salad	27
Salad with flowers	28
Fresh summer salad	29
Strawberry lentil salad	30
Pigeon peas salad	31
Avocado and papaya salad	32
Avocado haricot salad	33
chopped Mediterranean salad	34
Southwestern salad	35
Low-carb chicken salad	36
Avocado and tomato salad	37
Eggs with vegetable	38
Zucchini Omelet	39
Omelet with mushrooms	40
Simply omelet	41
Salad omelet wrap	42
Turmeric pancakes with leek	43
Minestrone	47
Mexican vegetable soup	48
Detox cabbage soup	49
Spring asparagus soup	50
Pea soup	51
Lentil and potato soup	52
Barley and vegetable soup	53
Chicken noodle soup	54
Detox potato turmeric soup	55
Yam and gungo soup	56
Overnight oats with apple and walnuts	60
Spicy kernels	61
Cherry yogurt popsicles	62
Vegan avocado dessert	63
Baked banana	64
Millet and pear muesli	65
Skyr with passion fruit sauce	66
Protein pancakes	67
Red dessert	68
Fruit quark with linseed oil	69
Quark dessert	70
Vegan sweet cherry bars	71
Quark pancakes with fruit	72
Potato goulash	76
Rosemary-roasted potatoes	77
Sweet potato pone	78
Scalloped potatoes	79
Kartoffel-blumenkohl-curry	80
Potato and cheesecake	81
Winter bowl with potato	83
Cottage cheese and potato toast	84
Sweet potato salad	85
Sauerkraut kumpir	86
Fried potato and asparagus pan	87
Sweet potato and carrot gratin	88
Peanut and sweet potato soup	89
Potato and radish salad	90
Aubergines	91

GOUT DIET COOKBOOK

What is Gout?

Gout describes a set of conditions with one common feature – the accumulation of uric acid inside the joints.

Uric acid is a product of the catabolic reaction of purine nucleotides, and it is a standard component of urine.

Generally speaking, gout affects the joints of the feet and hands, causing edema (i.e., swelling), pain, and reduced range of motion.
According to reports, gout affects 3.9% of the population in the United States; this translates to approximately 9.2 million people. (1)

The causes of gout

Gout stems from the buildup of uric acid in the bloodstream, which eventually leads to the leakage of this chemical into the joint capsules. (2) As a result, an inflammatory reaction sets in, producing the classic signs and symptoms of gout.

Researchers identified metabolic disorders, dehydration, and certain vascular diseases as potential triggers of uric acid accumulation. Additionally, medical conditions that affect the kidneys and thyroid also interfere with the body's ability to remove excess uric acid from the blood.

Other risk factors of gout include: (3)

Age – middle-aged men and postmenopausal women
Family history – having family members with gout increases the risk
Alcohol abuse – excessive alcohol consumption precipitates gout
Medication – diuretics, cyclosporine
Concurrent medical conditions – high blood pressure, thyroid disease, diabetes, kidney disease, and obstructive sleep apnea
Dietary choices – foods rich in gout-producing purines (e.g., some fish, organ meats, game meats)

The signs and symptoms of gout

Acute gout attacks present with a variety of symptoms that last between 3 to 10 days.

Classic symptoms include:
Pain
Edema
The warmth of the skin above the joint

Once the attack subsides, you will not experience any of these symptoms. Unfortunately, untreated gout can become chronic, especially when the triggering factor is still present. Moreover, hard lumps (i.e., tophi) can deposit around the skin, joints, and soft tissues, which permanently damages the structure of your joints. (4)

After pain treatment, to provide relief, the first therapy goal is to lower the levels of uric acids in the blood, which allows preventing new painful episodes (or at least a reduction in their frequency).

A careful and mindful diet can help reduce uric acid levels in the blood, and while it cannot be called a cure, it can effectively reduce the risk of recurrent gout attacks and slow the progression of joint damage. Parallel to the pharmacological intervention of medical relevance, the diet must be customized according to the patient's needs.

What kind of food is good and which to avoid

Nutrition plays a vital role in both the prevention and treatment of gout; for example, alcohol abuse or a diet that is too rich and careless often increases uric acids.

Foods that can trigger gout attacks

If you are susceptible to gout attacks, you need to avoid purine-producing foods. These foods typically contain more than 200 mg of purine per 3.5 ounces.

Here is a list of the significant purine-producing foods to avoid:

Fish: Herring, trout, mackerel, tuna, sardines, anchovies, haddock
Other seafood: Scallops, crab, shrimp, and roe
Organ meats: These include liver, kidneys, sweetbreads, and brain
Game meats: Examples include pheasant, veal, and venison, fatty meat broth or meat extracts, sausage, goose, duck, lard
Sugary beverages: Especially fruit juices and sugary sodas
Added sugars: honey, agave nectar, and high-fructose corn syrup
Yeasts: Nutritional yeast, brewer's yeast, and other yeast supplements
Alcohol specialty beer

A too restrictive diet also leads to a rise in uric acid concentration, derived from particular molecules' metabolism, called purines.

If you are overweight or obese, your diet should be moderately low-calorie to reach the desired weight gradually, but not excessively drastic to avoid causing a further increase in blood uric acid levels.

The general advice, beyond these first indications, are

Avoid prolonged fasting.
Avoid a diet too rich in fats and proteins, consequently avoiding or decreasing foods rich in purines (anchovies, brain, liver, kidneys, shrimp, sardines, ...).
Avoid alcohol consumption.
Drink plenty of water to prevent kidney stones from forming.
Consume copious amounts of fruits, vegetables, and whole grains, which provide healthy carbohydrates in complex form.

Following foods are good foods for GOUT diet:
plant foods: fruit, vegetables, nuts, seeds, including cereals, lean fish, chicken, turkey, skimmed milk, extra virgin olive oil, coffee, tea, and herbal teas.

Foods to consume with moderation:
mayonnaise, asparagus, peas, tomatoes, and spinach (limit to use these vegetables because of the suspect of relationship with the possibility of developing kidney stones, but a good intake of water allows their consumption), pork or beef (lean parts only), whole milk, dried fruit, simple sugars.

Another important trick is not to use too much fat when cooking, preferring approaches such as: steaming, boiling, plate, foil, sautéed.

If you want to consume a fry, you need to make sure that the oil temperature is high enough not to be absorbed by the food, but obviously, avoid fried foods in recent remission of an acute attack.

Instead of salt, use: garlic, onion, various spices, vinegar, lemon.

How to relieve your gout pain with food - homemade remedies

In this section, we will tackle some of the foods that improve the symptoms of gout.

Ginger

Researchers found that applying ginger to the joints can relieve pain induced by gout. (5)
In one laboratory study, researchers analyzed the effects of ginger supplementation on uric acid levels. The results showed that regular intake of ginger prevents hyperuricemia (i.e., elevated levels of uric acid in the blood). (6)

Here is what you need to do to apply ginger on the affected articulations:
Turn ginger into a paste by boiling water with one tablespoon of grated fresh ginger root
Soak a washcloth in the mixture
When it cools down, apply the washcloth to the affected joints for 15–30 minutes.
Do this at least once a day.

Cherries

According to one study, cherries (e.g., sour, sweet, red, black) effectively dampen inflammation induced by gout attacks. (7)
Researchers believe that cherries exert their anti-inflammatory and antioxidative effects, translating into pain relief and reduced swelling.

Magnesium

Low magnesium levels can often exacerbate gout attacks and similar conditions.
In a 2015 study, scientists found a correlation between adequate magnesium consumption and lower uric acid levels. Interestingly, these findings were only noted in men and not women. (8)

Nettle tea

Stinging nettle (Urtica dioica) is a potent remedy that addresses inflammation and pain.
In one study, nettle tea showed kidney-protecting properties that improve the clearance of uric acid. (9)
To prepare this tea, steep two tablespoons of dried nettle in some water and boil it.

Milk thistle seeds
Milk thistle improves the function of the liver and kidneys.
In one study, researchers found that this herb reduces uric acid levels even when patients have kidney failure. (10)

Hibiscus
Hibiscus is a traditional herb used as food, tea, or garden flower.
Adding hibiscus in a home remedy can relieve symptoms of gout by lowering the levels of uric acid. (11)

References

1-Singh, G., Lingala, B., & Mithal, A. (2019). Gout and hyperuricemia in the USA: prevalence and trends. Rheumatology (Oxford, England), 58(12), 2177–2180. https://doi.org/10.1093/rheumatology/kez196

2-Ragab, G., Elshahaly, M., & Bardin, T. (2017). Gout: An old disease in a new perspective– A review. Journal of advanced research, 8(5), 495-511.

3-Singh, J. A., Reddy, S. G., & Kundukulam, J. (2011). Risk factors for gout and prevention: a systematic review of the literature. Current opinion in rheumatology, 23(2), 192.

4-Ragab, G., Elshahaly, M., & Bardin, T. (2017). Gout: An old disease in a new perspective– A review. Journal of advanced research, 8(5), 495-511.

5-https://www.ijstr.org/final-print/oct2017/Effect-Of-Red-Ginger-Compress-To-Decrease-Scale-Of-Pain-Gout-Arthiris-Patients.pdf

6-http://www.journalijar.com/uploads/666_IJAR-7458.pdf

7-Singh, J. A., Bharat, A., & Edwards, N. L. (2015). An internet survey of common treatments used by patients with gout, including cherry extract and juice and other dietary supplements. Journal of clinical rheumatology: practical reports on rheumatic & musculoskeletal diseases, 21(4), 225.

8-Wang, Y. L., Zeng, C., Wei, J., Yang, T., Li, H., Deng, Z. H., ... & Lei, G. H. (2015). Association between dietary magnesium intake and hyperuricemia. PLoS One, 10(11), e0141079.

9-Salih, N. A. (2015). Effect of nettle (Urtica dioica) extracts on gentamicin-induced nephrotoxicity in male rabbits. Asian Pacific Journal of Tropical Biomedicine, 5(9), 756-760.

10-Karakuş, A., Değer, Y., & Yıldırım, S. (2017). Protective effect of Silybum marianum and Taraxacum officinale extracts against oxidative kidney injuries induced by carbon tetrachloride in rats. Renal failure, 39(1), 1-6.

11-Kuo, C. Y., Kao, E. S., Chan, K. C., Lee, H. J., Huang, T. F., & Wang, C. J. (2012). Hibiscus sabdariffa L. extracts reduce serum uric acid levels in oxonate-induced rats. Journal of Functional Foods, 4(1), 375-381.

TABLE

Food with moderate purine mg/100g

Beef chuck, filet, fore rib, entrecote, shoulder, roast beef	120
Bean dry white seed	128
soya dry seed dry	190
chicken breast	175
chicken for roasting	115
chicken legs with skin and bone	110
fish anchovy	239
fish cod	109
fish haddock	139
fish herring roe	190
fish mackerel	145
fish redfish	241
fish salmon	170
fish sole	131
fish eel smoked	78
crayfish	60
ham cooked	131
grape dried raisin	107
lentil dry seed	127
linseed	105
lobster	118
peas chick, dry garbanzo seed	109
poppy seed	170
rabbit meat average	132

Food with low purine mg/100gr

almond	37	corn sweet	52
apple	14	cress	28
apricot	73	crispbread	60
asparagus	23	cucumber	7
aubergine	21	currant red	17
avocado	19	date dried	35
banana	57	elderberry black	33
bean sprouts	80	endive	17
bean french string beans haricot	37	fenel leaves	14
beans french dried	45	fig dried	64
blueberry, huckleberry, bilberry	22	grape	27
bread white	14	kale	48
broccoli	81	kiwi	18
brussels sprouts	69	leek	74
cabbage red savoy	35	lettuce	13
cabbage white	22	lettuce lambs	38
carrot	17	melon cantelope	33
cauliflower	51	mushroom chanterelle	17
celeriac	30	nuts brazil	23
cheese brie	7	nuts hazelnut	37
cheese cheddar ceshire	6	nuts peanut	79
cheese cottage	9	nuts walnut	25
cheese edam	7	oats whole grain	94
cheese Limburger	32	olive marinated green	29
cherry morelly	18	onion	13
cherry sweet	7	orange	19
chicory	12	parsley leaf	57
Chinese leaves	21	pasta made with eggs	40
chives	67	pea pod and seed, green	84

Food with low purine mg/100gr

pea seed dry	95
peach	21
pear	12
peppers green	55
pineapple	19
plum	24
plum dried	64
potato	16
potato cooked with skin	18
pumpkin	44
radish	15
radishes	14
raspberry	18
rhubarb	12
rice white	26
rols bread	21
sauerkraut dripped off	16
sesame seeds	62
spinach	57
strawberry	21
tomato	11
yogurt 3.5 %fat	8

Reference: https://elevatehealthaz.com/wp-content/Purine%20Table.pdf

Many recipes in this cookbook mention using vegetable broth or vegetable soup. Here is the recipe for healthy vegetable broth with very low sodium.

VEGETABLE BROTH

Ingredients:

2 onions chopped
4 cloves garlic
3 carrots
4 celery stalks
5 sprigs of fresh thyme
1 bay leaf
1 small bunch of fresh parsley
½ small bunch of fresh basil leaf
1 tsp black peppercorns
1 medium leek (especially the green parts),
1 fennel,
1 tomato,
1 small bunch of fresh parsnip,
1 tbsp olive oil

Preparation:

Wash all vegetables. In a big pot, warm olive oil, add onions and stir for 2 minutes. Add all coarsely chopped vegetables and spices. Add water to cover vegetables and bring to a boil. When boiling, reduce the temperature to medium and simmer for 1 hour.

Let it cool for a while, and then drain the vegetables. You can use the vegetable soup clean and freeze it for later. If you want, you can blend all vegetables into the vegetable soup and freeze the smoothie soup in small glasses or ice cubes. The broth will have a mild taste if you add more water, depending on you. You can add or change any vegetable from the ingredients list but avoid potatoes and other starchy ones, zucchini, aubergine, beans.

You can roast the vegetables into the oven for one hour before using them as described in the recipe. Roast just hard vegetables, let the leaves boil, and the soup will be even more aromatic.

VEGETABLES

SALADS

Servings: 4

 Calories: 120

 ready in 50min

SPICY PLANTAINS

Ingredients:

2 firm-ripe plantains - a yellow one
2 spring onions finely chopped
1 fresh tomato chopped
1 red pepper thinly sliced
½ tsp of mild curry powder
1 tbsp rapeseed oil
the small stem of ginger about a tbsp peeled and finely chopped
scotch bonnet pepper to taste
approx 8 mg purine

Instructions:

Make an incision along the length of each plantain so it is easier to peel once cooked. Boil in water for 10-15 minutes until plantain can be easily pierced with a fork. Remove from water and leave to cool.

Heat the rapeseed oil in a large non-stick pan. Add the spring onion, red pepper, ginger, and tomato and cook gently for 8-10 minutes—season with black pepper to taste. Meanwhile, peel the plantains, discard the skin, and slice into discs about 1 inch thick. Transfer plantains to the pan and mix well. Serve as a starchy food with meat or fish and a portion of vegetables.

Servings: 10

Calories: 240

ready in 1 hour

SPICY BANANA BREAD

Ingredients:

3 ripe bananas - mashed
2 medium eggs
1 tsp baking powder
3 tsp mixed spice
1 tsp vanilla essence
3 tbsp caster sugar
¾ cup plain white flour
5 tbsp oats
approx 1,5 mg purine

Instructions:

Combine the eggs, spices, and banana in a large bowl and mix well. Sieve the flour and fold into the mixture, then add the oats.

Use fry light or vegetable oil to grease a baking tin or line with greaseproof paper. Pour in the mixture and level the surface.

Bake in the middle of the oven at 190 C/370 F for 34 - 40 minutes. Allow the bread to cool for 15 minutes and turn out onto a wire rack. Serve warm.

Servings: 8

Calories: 240

ready in 5 min

POPPYSEED SALAD

Ingredients:

Lettuce
Onion green
string beans
Acai berry
Citrus fruits
Grapes with no seeds
Avocado

For Dressing:
vinaigrette
3 tbsp of poppy seeds
Olive oil
salt pepper
approx 12 mg purine

Instructions:

Rinse the string beans. Wash and clean vegetables, cut onion green, lettuce, and avocado.
Mix all ingredients in a bowl.
Add two or three tbsps of dressing, and toss.

Servings: 4　　　 Calories: 56　　　 ready in 10min

SEAWEED SALAD

Ingredients:

2 tbsp grams white sesame seeds
1 cup grams fresh wakame seaweed
1 tbsp Lime juice
1 tsp of sugar
chili's (freshly ground)
2 tbsp sesame seed oil
approx 7 mg purine

Instructions:

In a dry skillet, toast sesame seeds until fragrant and light brown. Remove the skillet from the heat and set it aside to cool. Drain the seaweed after rinsing it.
Add the seaweed to a bowl with lime juice, sugar, and pepper. Mix the sesame seeds and oil, season with salt and pepper to taste, and serve.

Servings: 4

 Calories: 348

 ready in 25min

BREAD SALAD

Ingredients:

6 whole-grain baguette slices
3 tbsp olive oil
2 shallots
one garlic clove
2 tbsp pitted black olives
1 basil bunch
1 tbsp vinegar (white)
1 cup feta cheese
cayenne
 approx 13 mg purine

Instructions:

Cut the whole grain baguette into 1-inch cubes with a sharp knife.
Heat 1 tbsp olive oil in a skillet and toast the bread cubes for 5 minutes over medium heat. Put them aside.
Peel the shallots and garlic cloves. Chop the garlic and cut the shallots into fine circles. Cut the olives in half. Basil should be washed, dried, and finely chopped. Combine the prepared ingredients and the bread cubes in a mixing bowl, add remaining oil, pepper, vinegar, and crumble the feta on top. Serve the bread salad with olives on four plates.

Servings: 4

 Calories: 256

 ready in 25min

SPRING SALAD

Ingredients:

3 cups mixed salad (for example, loose-leaf lettuce, butterhead lettuce, Batavia, and radicchio)
1 onion
3 tbsp white wine vinegar,
4 tbsp extra virgin olive oil
chilies
half cup parmesan cheese (a piece)
daisies (to serve)
approx 12 mg purine

Instructions:

Wash the salad leaves, sort them, shake them dry, and cut them into bite-size bits. Peel the onion and thinly slice or dice. Combine vinegar and olive oil in a salad dressing shaker. Shake well. Add pepper to taste.

Mix the salad leaves with the onion and divide evenly among four plates. Sprinkle each dish with salad dressing. Serve the salad with shredded Parmesan and daisies sprinkled on top.

Servings: 4

Calories: 200

ready in 35min

PAPAYA SALAD

Ingredients:

1 ½ cup salsify
2 tbsp apple cider vinegar
1 ½ cup papaya (1 papaya)
1 chicory
½ cup radicchio
½ cup gorgonzola (45% fat in dry matter)
½ cup yogurt (3.5% fat)
1 tbsp olive oil
pepper
4 tbsp grainy oat flakes
1 handful basil (5 g)
approx 27 mg purine

Instructions:

Thoroughly clean salsify, peel and cut into pieces approx. 1 inch in size. Boil them in salted water with 1 tbsp of apple cider vinegar for 15 minutes. Then drain, rinse with cold water, and set aside.
In the meantime, peel and core the papaya and cut it into fine strips. Wash and clean the chicory and radicchio and cut them into fine strips.
Put the Gorgonzola with yogurt, olive oil, and 1 tbsp apple cider vinegar in a tall container and puree finely with a hand blender, adding a little water if necessary. Season to taste with salt and pepper.
Roast the oatmeal in a hot pan without fat over medium heat for 3-4 minutes. Wash the basil, shake dry and cut into fine strips.
Arrange salsify, papaya, chicory, and radicchio on four plates, pour the dressing over them and sprinkle with oat flakes and basil strips

Servings: 2
 Calories: 565
 ready in 25min

STRAWBERRY DRESSING SALAD

Ingredients:

3 eggs
½ cup of lamb's lettuce
1 cup cucumber
radish bunch
12 spring onions, fretted
½ cup strawberries (or other seasonally available fruit)
2 tbsp olive oil
1 tbsp balsamic vinaigrette
salt, cayenne
thyme, dried
½ cup Sheep cheese (45 percent fat in dry matter)
2 pcs whole grain bread
approx 15 mg purine

Instructions:

Boil eggs for about 6 minutes, then set aside to cool.
Clean, wash and spin dry the lamb's lettuce. Cucumber, radishes, and spring onions should be cleaned, washed, and sliced. Strawberries should be cleaned and washed before being cut into fine cubes.
Combine the strawberries, olive oil, and vinegar in a mixing bowl—season to taste with salt, pepper, and thyme.
Peel and cut the eggs in half. Crumble the sheep's cheese. Combine the lettuce, cucumber, radish slices, spring onions, and feta cheese in a salad bowl. Serve the salad with the eggs on top, drizzled with the dressing, and bread on the side.

Servings: 4

Calories: 372

ready in 10min

SALAD WITH FLOWERS

Ingredients:

4 cups spring greens (mixed) (arugula, sorrel, young dandelion, watercress, etc.)
1 3/4 cup cheese, diced (cheddar, pepper jack, gouda; may substitute cheese of your choosing)
2 tbsp. vinegar (fruit)
1 tbsp lemon
5 tbsp. extra virgin olive oil
Black pepper freshly ground blossoms that are edible (such as pansies; dandelions, and daisies)
approx 19 mg purine

Instructions:

Clean, wash and rinse the mixed greens. Divide them into four salad bowls, and sprinkle diced cheese over the top of each salad bowl.
Whisk the vinegar, lemon juice, oil, salt, and pepper in a small mixing bowl until well combined. Drizzle over salad and add new edible flowers for a finishing touch.

Servings: 4

Calories: 166

ready in 40min

FRESH SUMMER SALAD

Ingredients:

4 cups white asparagus (trimmed)
a pot of hot water
1 tsp butter
2 lemons (juice)
2 2/3 cup strawberries, chopped
3 tbsp balsamic vinegar (white)
2 tbsp olive oil (extra virgin)
2 tbsp lemon juice
peppers, freshly ground
as finishing touch, basil (herb)
arugula
approx 18 mg purine

Instructions:

Cut the ends off the asparagus stalks and peel them.
Boil water with asparagus, butter, and lemon juice until soft asparagus. Drain the asparagus and rinse it in cold water before draining it again.
Chop the asparagus coarsely and combine it with the strawberries.
Combine the vinegar, oil, lemon juice, salt, and pepper to taste in a mixing bowl.
Mix the asparagus and strawberries with the dressing, divide among serving plates.
Serve with basil and rocket on the side.

Servings: 4

Calories: 383

ready in 35min

STRAWBERRY LENTIL SALAD

Ingredients:

1 cup lentils
1 cup edamame
2 rhubarb sticks (young)
1 cup strawberries,
1 cup Snow peas,
1 tbsp sesame seed oil
2 tbsp lemon juice
bunch of basil
½ cup bocconcini (small fresh mozzarella balls)
approx 90 mg purine

Instructions:

Boil the lentils until they are soft, as directed on the packet. Drain, set it aside, and let it cool.
Boil the edamame for 5 minutes in salted water. Drain and cool before removing the edamame from the pods.
Prepare the rhubarb and strawberries by washing, cleaning, and slicing them.
Snow peas should be washed, cleaned, and cut in half diagonally.
Combine sesame oil, lemon juice, salt, and pepper in a large mixing bowl.
Basil should be washed, dried, and coarsely chopped.
Add all ingredients together with the dressing and divide among four bowls. Distribute the mozzarella among the bowls.

Servings: 4 Calories: 130 ready in 40min

PIGEON PEAS SALAD

Ingredients:

2 cups green pigeon peas
1 cup of sweetcorn in unsalted water drained
2 medium carrots peeled and grated
2 spring onions finely chopped

for the sauce:
3 tbsp olive oil
1 tbsp balsamic vinegar
1 tiny chili seeds removed, finely chopped
1 tsp minced garlic
juice of 1 lime
a handful of parsley roughly chopped
approx 58 mg purine

Instructions:

Use dried peas, boil them for about 30 minutes. Drain and leave to cool.
If you use canned peas: empty the contents into a colander. Rinse with cold water and drain well.
Combine all ingredients for the dressing in a large bowl, season with black pepper to taste. Pour the sauce over the peas, sweet corn, and grated carrot, mixing well. Add chopped spring onions to garnish.

Servings: 4

Calories: 380

ready in 15min

AVOCADO AND PAPAYA SALAD

Ingredients:

4 avocado
4 papayas peeled, halved, and seeded
2 limes zested and juiced
2 baby gem lettuces
1 small red onion finely diced
1 handful of cherry tomatoes halved
1 clove garlic minced
½ tsp freshly ground black pepper
½ tsp cayenne pepper
¼ cup olive oil
approx 17 mg purine

Instructions:

Slice the avocado lengthwise into ½ inch slices. Slice the papaya width-wise into ½ inch slices, drizzle with the juice of 1 lime immediately.
Arrange slices overlapping and alternating on a bed of baby gem lettuce, then add the cherry tomatoes and onions.

In a small bowl, combine remaining ingredients, mix well, spoon over the salad and serve immediately.

Servings: 4

 Calories: 503

 ready in 10 min

AVOCADO HARICOT SALAD

Ingredients:

Dressing:
2 tbsp olive oil
¼ cup lime juice
2 tsp cumin
2 tsp chili powder
1 tsp salt
1 tsp pepper
Salad:
¼ cup fresh cilantro, chopped
2 cups haricot beans, drained, rinsed
1 cucumber, chopped, quartered
5 cherry tomatoes halved
1 onion, chopped
1 avocado, diced
⅓ cup carrot, shredded
approx 25 mg purine

Instructions:

For the dressing: combine dressing ingredients in a small bowl. Whisk together until mixed thoroughly.
Combine beans, cucumber, tomatoes, onion, avocado, carrots, and dressing in a large bowl. Toss together until evenly combined.

Servings: 4

Calories: 208

ready in 15 min

CHOPPED MEDITERRANEAN SALAD

Ingredients:

2 cucumbers
4 tomatoes
1 red onion
½ cup feta cheese
2 tbsp olive oil
2 tbsp red wine vinegar
salt,
black pepper, to taste
1 tbsp lemon juice
1 cup olive
approx 10 mg purine

Instructions:

Peel the cucumbers. Cut into discs, and then quarter the discs. Place in a large salad bowl.

Cut tomatoes into quarters, lengthwise, and then rotate and cut into large chunks. Add to the salad bowl.

Cut the red onion in half, removing the skin, stem, and bottom. Thinly slice and add to the bowl.

Add the feta cheese, olive oil, red wine vinegar, salt, pepper, lemon juice, and olives to the salad bowl and toss gently.

Servings: 5

 Calories: 342

 ready in 15mn

SOUTHWESTERN SALAD

Ingredients:

Dressing:
1 avocado, halved
1 clove garlic
½ tsp salt
½ tsp pepper
2 tbsp olive oil
1 tbsp fresh cilantro
1 lime, juiced
Salad:
1 head lettuce, chopped
1 cup bell pepper, chopped
¼ cup fresh cilantro
1 cup black beans
½ cup red onion, chopped
1 cup corn
¼ cup scallion
¾ cup tomato, chopped
approx 18 mg purine

Instructions:

Add all dressing ingredients to a blender, blend until smooth.
Add lettuce, peppers, cilantro, beans, onion, corn, green onion, and tomatoes in a large bowl.
Top with prepared dressing; toss.

Servings: 4

 Calories: 250

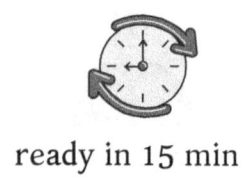 ready in 15 min

LOW-CARB CHICKEN SALAD

Ingredients:

⅔ cup greek yogurt low fat
1 tbsp lime juice
pepper, to taste
⅛ tsp chili powder
1 avocado, cubed, divided
2 chicken breasts, cooked and shredded
1 stalk celery, diced
2 tbsp red onion, diced
salt
bread, low-carb, for serving, optional
fresh cilantro leaf for garnish
approx 40 mg purine

Instructions:

In a blender or food processor, combine the yogurt, lime juice, pepper, and chili powder, add ½ of the avocado and blend until creamy.

Combine the chicken, yogurt sauce, celery, the remaining ½ avocado, onion, and salt in a medium bowl. Mix until well combined.

Serve on the low-carb bread and garnish with cilantro.

Servings: 2

Calories: 161

ready in 15 min

AVOCADO AND TOMATO SALAD

Ingredients:

1 avocado, diced
1 cup cherry tomato, finely chopped
¼ medium red onion, thinly sliced
½ lime, juiced
salt, to taste
2 tbsps fresh parsley, chopped
bunch of cashews
approx 20 mg purine

Instructions:

Combine all ingredients in a bowl and gently stir.

Servings: 6

 Calories: 170

 ready in 15min

EGGS WITH VEGETABLE

Ingredients:

8 large eggs
1/2 yellow onion chopped
1/2 cup carrots chunk chopped and steamed
1/4 cup green peas
1/2 cup green bell pepper chopped
1/4 cup bean sprouts cut in half
1 tbsp light soy sauce
3 tbsp sesame oil divided
approx 46 mg purine

Instructions:

Add the eggs, onion, carrots, peas, bell pepper, bean sprouts, and soy sauce together in a bowl and whisk to combine.

In a large skillet, heat 1 tsp of sesame oil at a time for each pancake you fry on medium heat.

Add about 1/3 cup of mixture per pancake and fry for 3-4 minutes on the first one and 1-2 minutes on the other side

Servings: 2

Calories: 581

ready in 15min

ZUCCHINI OMELETTE

Ingredients:

1 cup - one large zucchini
2 red onions
1 red pepper
6 eggs
1 cup milk (1.5 percent fat)
cumin
paprika powder
2 tbsp of extra virgin olive oil
½ cup soft goat cheese (45 percent fat in dry matter)
½ cup arugula
approx 30 mg purine

Instructions:

Clean and wash the zucchini, halved lengthwise, and cut into slices. Peel and halve the onions and cut them into strips. Halve, core, wash and cut the pepper into strips.

Whisk eggs with milk, season with salt, pepper, and paprika powder.

Heat 1 tbsp of oil in a pan and fry half of the vegetables for about 5 minutes. Add half of the egg-milk and let it set. Fry a second a omelet the same way.

Cut the cheese into slices. Wash the rocket and shake dry. Spread the goat cheese and rocket on the omelets, slide out of the pan and serve.

Servings: 4

Calories: 304

ready in 25 min

OMELETTE WITH MUSHROOMS

Ingredients:

1 cup brown mushrooms
1 shallot
2 tbsps of extra virgin olive oil
cumin
8 eggs
half cup milk (1.5 percent fat)
1 pinch turmeric powder
3 slices cheddar cheese
half bunch chervil
approx 28 mg purine

Instructions:

Clean the mushrooms and cut them into slices. Peel and finely dice shallots. Heat 1 tbsp of olive oil in a pan. Add mushrooms and shallots and sauté for 3-4 minutes over medium heat. Season with salt and pepper, remove from the pan, and set aside. Whisk eggs with milk—season with one pinch of turmeric, salt, and pepper. Brush a coated pan with a bit of oil, add 1/4 of the egg mixture and swirl to distribute it evenly. Top with 1/4 of the fried mushrooms. Cook the omelet over medium heat for 2-3 minutes and brown lightly. Pluck 1/4 of the Cheddar into pieces, cover the omelet with it, slide out of the pan and keep warm in the preheated oven at 80 ° C / 170 F. Bake three more omelets in the same way. Wash the chervil, shake dry and pluck the leaves. Garnish each omelet with pepper and chervil tips and serve.

Servings: 4

 Calories: 280

 ready in 20 min

SIMPLY OMELET

Ingredients:

1 tbsp olive oil (plus more for the omelets)
½ cup bell pepper
½ cup sliced cremini or button mushrooms
½ cup diced onion
taste with black pepper and salt
8 eggs
2 tbsp milk (low fat)
½ cup sharp shredded Cheddar
approx 28 mg purine

Instructions:

In a medium sauté pan, heat the olive oil on medium. Add onion and mushrooms and fry for 7 minutes, until the bell pepper, mushrooms, and onions are softened and lightly browned. Season with salt and pepper
In a mixing bowl, whisk together the eggs and milk until smooth.
In a small non-stick skillet, heat the oil over medium-high heat.
Pour one-quarter of the eggs into the pan and, as soon as they start to set, scrape the egg from the bottom with a wooden spoon, working from one hand to the other (like you were scrambling eggs).
When the egg is almost over, stop scraping and scatter a quarter of the cheese and a quarter of the vegetable mixture around the omelet. Fold the egg over on itself with a spatula. Transfer the omelet to a warm plate by sliding it out of the pan. Create four omelets this way.

Servings: 6

 Calories: 170

 ready in 15min

SALAD OMELETTE WRAP

Ingredients:

4 lettuce leaves
½ cup Carrots,
Black pepper, freshly ground

The omelet's Ingredients
4 eggs
2 tbsp butter
approx 18 mg purine

Instructions:

Wash the lettuce leaves and cut them into thin strips after draining them. Carrots should be peeled and sliced thinly.

In a mixing bowl, beat the eggs. In an 8-inch (20-cm) skillet, melt one tbsp of butter and add half of the egg mixture. Remove the omelet from the skillet until the egg has set, and repeat with the remaining egg.

To make a wrap, place the omelets on a tray, top with lettuce strips and carrots, season with salt and pepper, and roll-up. Serve by slicing in half on the diagonal.

Servings: 4　　 Calories: 320　　 ready in 40min

TURMERIC PANCAKES WITH LEEK

Ingredients:

½ cup wholemeal spelled flour
1 cup milk
2 eggs
salt
1 tsp turmeric powder
1 cup leek (1 small stick)
1 zucchini
1 apple
3 tbsp rapeseed oil
½ cup cream cheese (45% fat in dry matter)
pepper
¼ tsp ground caraway seeds
¼ tsp dried marjoram
approx 28 mg purine

Instructions:

Mix flour with milk, eggs, 2–4 tbsps of water, salt, and turmeric powder to form a smooth dough and leave to swell for 10 minutes. In the meantime, clean and wash the leek and courgette and cut them into thin rings and pieces. Wash the apple, cut in half, core, and cut into small pieces. Heat 1 tbsp of oil in a pan. Sauté the leek and zucchini in it over medium heat for 5 minutes. Add apple and sauté for 3 minutes. Add the cream cheese and 3–4 tbsps of water and stir until creamy. Season with salt, pepper, caraway seeds, and marjoram.
For the pancakes, spread a large pan with 1 tsp of oil each. Pour in 1 ladle of the egg mix and fry on medium heat for 2–3 minutes on each side. Fill the pancakes with vegetables and serve.

SOUPS

Servings: 6

Calories: 205

ready in 1 hour

MINESTRONE (VEGETABLE SOUP)

Ingredients:
5 tbsp extra virgin olive oil
1 white onion, finely chopped
1 garlic clove, finely chopped
2 peeled and cubed potatoes (or sweet potatoes)
1 cup peeled and cubed pumpkin
2 thickly cut carrots
1 thickly cut celery stalk
1 small head of broccoli, cut into small pieces
1 cubed zucchini
1 finely chopped leek
1 cup peas (frozen)
Water (1.5 liters) (or vegetable stock)
1 cup vegetable broth
a handful of vermicelli rice (or another small pasta shape)
black pepper, freshly ground
a few finely chopped new basil leaves
Grated Parmesan cheese is an optional topping.
approx 28 mg purine

Instructions:
Heat the extra virgin olive oil in a large pot over low heat, add the onion and garlic, cook for 3 minutes or until the onion is translucent.
Add all vegetables, starting with the hard ones (carrots, potatoes, pumpkin), then the softer ones (except the frozen peas), and combine well.
Boil the water, and vegetable broth, reduce to low heat and gently simmer for 30 minutes. Ten minutes before the cooking time, add the frozen peas.
Boil for another minute after adding the rice vermicelli. If using pasta, cook it in the soup until al dente (about 10 minutes) or as directed on the package.
Take the pan from the heat, season with salt and pepper, and whisk in the basil leaves. Serve in individual bowls with parmesan cheese and garlic bread.

Servings: 6

Calories: 154

ready in 1 hour

MEXICAN VEGETABLE SOUP

Ingredients:
1 1/2 cup yellow onion, chopped
1 1/2 tbsp extra virgin olive oil
2 garlic cloves, minced
5 cups vegetable broth (low sodium)
1 1/2 cans diced tomatoes with green chilies
1 3/4 cup zucchini (chopped)
Optional: 1 ¼ cup diced green beans
1 diced red bell pepper
1 tsp oregano (dried) (Mexican oregano if you have it)
1 tsp cumin powder
1 3/4 cup frozen corn or canned hominy, drained and rinsed
2 tbsp lime juice
1/2 cup cilantro, chopped
approx 38 mg purine

Instructions:
In a large pot, heat the olive oil over medium-high heat. Add the onions and carrots, cook for 3 minutes, and add garlic and cook for another minute. Season with salt and pepper, add the vegetable broth, onions, zucchini, green beans, bell pepper, oregano, and cumin. Bring to a boil, then reduce to medium-low heat, cover, and boil until the vegetables are tender, around 20 minutes.
Boil until the corn is cooked through, stirring in the lime juice and cilantro. Heat the dish before serving.

Servings: 6

 Calories: 62

 ready in 30 min

DETOX CABBAGE SOUP

Ingredients:

1/2 cabbage head
a total of 6 celery stalks
1 onion, big
1 bell pepper, green
5 cloves of garlic
Optional: 1/2 tsp red pepper flakes
1 tbsp oregano
1 cups vegetable stock
salt and pepper to taste
approx 22 mg purine

Instructions:

In a big pot over medium-high heat, warm some oil.
Fry the onions, celery, and peppers until they are translucent, around 5 minutes.
Season with salt and pepper, then add the red pepper flakes and oregano.
Add garlic and roast, constantly stirring until the garlic is fragrant.
Add the chicken stock and cabbage.
Cook until the cabbage is tender, about 15 minutes.

Servings: 4

 Calories: 101

 ready in 40min

SPRING ASPARAGUS SOUP

Ingredients:

2 1/2 cups sliced asparagus,
2 tsp coconut butter
3 shallots, chopped
1/2 cup red potatoes, chopped
3 cups vegetable broth
8 asparagus spears (halved, for garnish)
approx 20 mg purine

Instructions:

Sauté the asparagus spears for 30 seconds in 1/2 of the coconut butter and set aside for garnish.

In a deep non-stick pan, melt the remaining coconut butter, add the shallots and potatoes and cook for 3 to 4 minutes.

Pour in 2 cups vegetable stock, stir well, and cook until the potatoes are soft. Stir in the asparagus and cook for a few minutes more. Allow cooling.

Puree the mixture in a mixer until it is smooth.

Return the puree to the pan, season with salt and pepper, and add the remaining vegetable stock. Bring to a boil.

Garnish with sautéed asparagus spears and serve immediately.

Servings: 2

Calories: 533

ready in 14min

PEA SOUP

Ingredients:

1 shallot
1 garlic clove
2 tbsp olive oil
1 cup peas (frozen)
1 cup vegetable broth
4 dill stems
½ cup feta cheese
½ cup whipped cream
Chili flakes (optional)
1 tbsp black sesame seeds
approx 50 mg purine

Instructions:

Peel the garlic and shallot. Heat 1 tbsp of oil and sauté shallots and garlic for 3 minutes over medium heat in a saucepan. Cook for another 3 minutes after adding the peas. After that, add the vegetable stock and cook for 5 minutes. Meanwhile, wash and dry the dill before plucking it into small bits. Using your hands, crumble the feta cheese.

Next, pour the cream and finely puree the soup with half of the dill using a hand blender: salt, pepper, and chili flakes to taste in the pea soup. Fill two bowls with the remaining dill, feta, and sesame seeds, and drizzle with the remaining oil.

Servings: 4

 Calories: 351

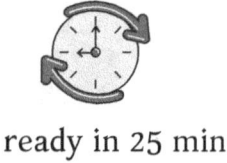 ready in 25 min

LENTIL AND POTATO SOUP

Ingredients:

3 carrots
1 cup potatoes
2 tbsp olive oil
½ cup red lentil
2 tbsp turmeric powder
4 cups vegetable broth
1 tbsp Tomato paste
cayenne
2 tbsp whipped cream
2 slices wholemeal sourdough bread
1 handful basil fresh
approx 50 mg purine

Instructions:

Peel and cut the carrots and potatoes into small cubes after cleaning them. In a saucepan, heat 1 tbsp of oil for 4 minutes over medium heat, sauté the carrots and potatoes in it.

Cook for 2 minutes after adding the lentils and turmeric.

Season with salt and pepper after adding the vegetable stock and tomato paste.

Boil the soup for about 15 minutes over low heat. Using a hand blender, puree in cream.

Dice bread slices at the same time. In a separate pan, heat the remaining oil. Over medium heat, toast the bread cubes for 5 minutes or until golden brown.

Clean the basil leaves by shaking them dry and plucking the leaves. Fill bowls halfway with broth, drizzle with cream, and top with bread cubes and basil.

Servings: 6

 Calories: 200

 ready in 30 min

BARLEY AND VEGETABLE SOUP

Ingredients:

3/4 cup pearl barley
4 cups vegetable stock
2 tbsp. extra-virgin olive oil
1 1/2 cup onion crumbled
1 cup carrots, chopped
1 celery stalk, chopped
1 cup mushrooms, thinly sliced
parsley (half bunch)
approx 30 mg purine

Instructions:

Add the barley with 3 cups vegetable stock in a saucepan.
Over medium heat, boil, cover for 1 hour or until the liquid is absorbed.
Meanwhile, in a large pot, heat the olive oil and add the onion, carrots, celery, and mushrooms.
Cook, covered, for 5 minutes, or until the vegetables soften.
Add remaining vegetable stock and cover and cook for 30 minutes
Cook for another 5 minutes with the barley.
Season to taste with salt and serve in bowls.
Garnish with fresh parsley chopped on top.

Servings: 8

Calories: 160

ready in 40min

CHICKEN NOODLE SOUP

Ingredients:

1 ½ cup long carrots, sliced
1 ½ cup long celery stalks
1 cup finely diced yellow onion
3 minced garlic cloves about a tbsp
2 ½ cups red potatoes, cubed into 1/2-inch cubes
6 to 7 cups of water
2 vegan bouillon cubes
1 tbsp thyme (dried)
2 cups brown spiral noodles
fresh parsley and lemon juice as an optional for garnish
approx 22 mg purine

Instructions:

Prepare all vegetables and spices and set them aside.
In a large pot, boil 6 cups of water, then add the bouillon cubes, thyme, salt, whisking to dissolve.
Add in a pot all vegetables (carrots, celery, onion, garlic, and potatoes) and spices. Bring to a boil, stirring constantly. When the water boils, reduce to low heat, cover, cook for around 10 minutes, or until the carrots and potatoes are tender but not thoroughly cooked. Add pasta and
return to a boil over medium-high heat for another 10 min or until the pasta is tender but firm. Check for salt and add a nice grind of freshly ground black pepper.
Before eating, garnish with freshly chopped parsley and a squeeze of lemon juice.

Servings: 5

Calories: 342

ready in 25min

DETOX POTATO TUMERIC SOUP

Ingredients:

4 big shallots
1 tbsp coconut oil
1/4 cup ginger, chopped
4 peeled garlic cloves, smashed with the side of a knife
1 big peeled and diced sweet potato
2 big carrots, peeled and chopped
1 tsp of turmeric
cayenne pepper + 1/2 tsp black pepper
4 cups vegetable stock
6 tbsp almond butter
1 coconut milk can (15 oz.)
1 Lemon juice
approx 70 mg purine

Instructions:

Add the coconut oil to a large pot over medium-high heat. Add the shallots and let them fry for 3-4 minutes. Add the garlic and ginger and fry for one more minute. Add the sweet potato, carrots, turmeric, sea salt, black pepper, and cayenne and stir the pot for about 30 seconds.
Add the stock to the pot and boil. Reduce the heat to medium and simmer for 10 minutes, or until the vegetables are soft. Transfer the soup to your blender, add the almond butter, and blend until smooth. Pour the soup back into the pot, add the coconut milk and lime juice, and heat through.

Servings: 6

Calories: 230

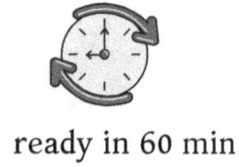
ready in 60 min

YAM AND GUNGO SOUP

Ingredients:

2 cups yams peeled and cubed
2 cups pigeon peas
70 oz water
2 cloves garlic crushed
2 stalks of spring onion
1 large green pepper
1 whole scotch bonnet of chili
3 sprigs of thyme
6 whole pimentos
approx 25 mg purine

Instructions:

Peel, then chop the yams into medium-sized chunks.
Finely chop the pimentos, garlic, and onion.
Boil the peas and yams until almost cooked for about 20 minutes.
Add all other ingredients and simmer for about 30 minutes until the broth thickens.

DESSERTS

Servings: 2   Calories: 426   ready in 15 min 12 hour

OVERNIGHT OATS WITH APPLE AND WALNUTS

Ingredients:
1 tsp cinnamon, salt
3 tbsp buckwheat flakes
1 cup milk (3.5 percent fat)
1 tbsp of applesauce (no added sugar)
2 tbsp chia seeds
1 apple
1 tbsp maple syrup
2 tbsp walnut kernels
approx 22 mg purine

Instructions:
Mix the buckwheat flakes with a pinch of salt and cinnamon. Stir in the milk, applesauce, and 1 tbsp chia seeds, then chill for at least 2 hours, preferably overnight.
The following day, wash, fifth, and core the apple. One half should be cut into fine wedges, while the other half should be cut into cubes. In a saucepan, combine the apple cubes and the remaining cinnamon; heat and allow to caramelize for 2-3 minutes.
Meanwhile, coarsely chop the walnuts. In two bowls or sealable glasses, place overnight oats. Arrange apple wedges, caramelized apple blocks, and walnuts on top, spread the remaining chia seeds, and cover oats with apple and walnuts.

Servings: 16

 Calories: 177

 Ready in 10 min

SPICY KERNELS

Ingredients:

¼ tsp powdered cloves
¼ tsp cardamom powder
¼ tsp cinnamon
1 cup Almond kernels
1 cup Cashew nuts
3 tbsp coconut oil (liquid)
4 tbsp sugar
approx 10 mg purine

Instructions:

Spread the kernels on a baking sheet lined with baking paper and roast for around 10 minutes at 200°C / 400 F in a preheated oven.
Remove from the oven and set aside to cool for 10 minutes.
Combine the spices in a bowl with the almonds, cashew nuts, coconut oil, sugar, kernels, and spice mixture. Fill a glass with a lid with 50 g of each and package it as a gift.

Servings: 6

Calories: 132

Ready in 20 min

CHERRY YOGURT POPSICLES

Ingredients:

1 ½ cup greek yogurt
1 cup organic lime (zest and juice)
½ cup cherries (fresh)
1 tbsp powdered birch sugar
approx 12 mg purine

Instructions:

Using a hand blender, puree the cherries with powdered birch sugar as finely as possible.

Strain through a fine sieve and combine yogurt, lime zest, and juice in a mixing bowl.

Pour the mixture into six ice cream molds and freeze. Allow for 1 hour of freezing time, then insert wooden handles and freeze for another 3 hours. To serve, remove the ice from the molds. Fresh cherries should be washed and arranged on a tart dish as desired before decorating ice cream.

Servings: 8

 Calories: 116

 Ready in 10min

VEGAN AVOCADO DESSERT

Ingredients:

1 vanilla bean
1/4 cup cocoa powder (unsweetened)
1 cup freshly squeezed orange juice
1 orange with its zest
1 tbsp sugar de coco
1 tbsp cocoa nibs
approx 8 mg purine

Instructions:

Scoop avocado flesh into a blender with a spoon, then add vanilla bean seeds.
Combine the cocoa powder, orange juice, orange zest, coconut sugar, and salt in a large mixing bowl. Blend until smooth, scraping down the sides of the blender to get every last drop.
The texture should be silky and creamy. Add more orange juice or a splash of water if necessary.
Divide pudding among 8 4-6 oz. Ramekins or small bowls and chill until slightly firm, at least 2 hours.
Sprinkle with cocoa nibs and cover; chill until ready to serve!

Servings: 4

 Calories: 268

 Ready in 20min

BAKED BANANA

Ingredients:

2 cups ripe bananas (four ripe bananas)
1 cup skyr
1 tbsp of linseed oil
4 tbsp almond kernels, grated
1 tbsp maple syrup
approx 20 mg purine

Instructions:

Wash the bananas without peeling them, pat them dry, and put them on an oven shelf. Bake for around 10 minutes at 200°C / 390 F in a preheated oven until the shell is evenly black.
Meanwhile, cut the vanilla pod half lengthwise and scrape the pulp out with a knife. Blend the skyr and linseed oil until smooth. For 3 minutes, roast the almonds in a hot pan without fat over medium heat.
Remove the bananas from the oven. Remove the top half of the peel from the hot fruits and set aside. Distribute the skyr among four plates and top with the bananas. Serve with a drizzle of maple syrup and a sprinkling of almonds.

Servings: 2

 Calories: 472

 Ready in 20min

MILLET AND PEAR MUESLI

Ingredients:

½ cup millet
1 cup pears (2 pears)
3 tbsp walnut kernels
1 cup curd milk (1.5% fat)
1 tbsp liquid honey
1 pinch cinnamon
approx 55 mg purine

Instructions:

Put the millet in a saucepan with twice the amount of water, boil, and let it swell over low heat for about 10 minutes.
In the meantime, wash the pears, rub dry, quarter, core, and dice.
Roughly chop the walnut kernels with a large knife or a lightning chopper.
Transfer the millet to a bowl and let it cool down a bit, stirring occasionally.
Mix the curd, honey, and cinnamon. Mix in the diced pear and millet. Sprinkle the muesli with the walnuts and serve.

Servings: 4

 Calories: 238

 Ready in 20min

SKYR WITH PASSION FRUIT SAUCE

Ingredients:

2 cups skyr
1 tbsp agave syrup
6 passion fruit
1 tsp cornstarch
1 large oranges
1 tbsp honey
3 tbsp almond kernels
approx 15 mg purine

Instructions:

Mix the skyr with agave syrup and place it in the refrigerator. In the meantime, halve the passion fruit for the sauce, remove the pulp and mix with the cornstarch.

Squeeze the orange. Simmer the juice with passion fruit mixture and honey for about 3-4 minutes while stirring over low heat. Let the thickened passion fruit sauce cool for about 5 minutes.

In the meantime, roughly chop the almonds. Divide the skyr among four plates, smooth out a little, cover with the sauce and sprinkle with the almonds

Servings: 2   Calories: 416   Ready in 25min

PROTEIN PANCAKES

Ingredients:

2 tbsp almond flour
2 tbsp spelled flour
2 tbsp Quark (20 % fat)
1 tbsp baking powder (tartar)
Cinnamon, 1 pinch
1 tsp powdered vanilla
¼ cup Milk,
4 tbsp rapeseed oil
1 tbsp almonds (toasted)
2 tbsp Blueberries (60 g)
1 tbsp maple syrup (optional)
1 tbsp butter made from almonds
approx 18 mg purine

Instructions:

Whisk the eggs, almond flour, spelled flour, quark, baking powder, cinnamon, vanilla powder, and milk in a big mixing bowl. Add a splash of milk if the batter is too stiff.

In a non-stick pan, heat 2 tbsp of oil, pour 1 tbsp of batter into each pan, and bake 4–6 pancakes for 3–4 minutes on both sides over medium heat.

Toast the almond slivers for 2-3 minutes in a hot, non-stick skillet over medium heat.

Blueberries should be washed and dried before being used. Garnish the pancakes with berries, almond butter, maple syrup, and sliced almonds on top, and serve.

Servings: 4

Calories: 507

Ready in 30min

RED DESSERT

Ingredients:

For the Red cream;
2 ½ cups guava nectar
⅓ cup of sugar
a quarter tsp of cinnamon
⅛ tsp nutmeg
1/4 cup tapioca starch (quick-cooking)
1/2 gallon of water
1 tsp extract de Vanille

To make the Vanilla Cream;
1/2 gallon whole milk
1/2 cup lower fat cream
1 bean of vanilla
3 big yolks of eggs
1 tsp of sugar
approx 14 mg purine

Instructions:

For the Red cream: Bring guava nectar and sugar to a boil in a medium saucepan. Add the salt, cinnamon, and nutmeg and mix well. Mix the water and fast-cooking tapioca in a small pot. Gradually pour the tapioca mixture into the saucepan, stirring constantly. Bring to a boil once more, continuously stirring. When the tapioca grains are transparent, remove them from the heat. It should take about 13 minutes to complete this task. Add the vanilla extract and mix well. Let it cool.

To make the vanilla cream: Mix milk and cream in a medium saucepan. Scrape the seeds from the vanilla bean into the milk mixture, add the split vanilla bean to the milk. Bring the milk mixture to a low boil, then turn off the fire. Take out the vanilla bean pods.
In a medium mixing cup, whisk together the egg yolks and sugar. Whisk the hot milk mixture into the yolk mixture gradually. Return the custard to the saucepan and cook, constantly stirring, over low heat until it thickens. This will take about 5 minutes (do not boil). Pour the sauce into a pot, cover it, and keep it in the refrigerator until ready to use.
Fill the glass and combine both creams.

Servings: 3

Calories: 349

Ready in 10min

FRUIT QUARK WITH LINSEED OIL

Ingredients:

3 tbsp low-fat quark
3 tbsp milk (1.5 percent fat)
2 tbsp organic cold-pressed linseed oil
1 tbsp lemon juice
1 handful of your favorite fruit (banana, raspberries, or strawberries)
1 tbsp flax seeds, crushed (or almond slivers)
1 tsp honey (at will)
approx 12 mg purine

Instructions:

In a blender or hand blender, thoroughly combine all ingredients except the fruit.
To finish, chop the fruit into bite-size pieces and sprinkle with flax seeds or almond slivers. Combine the quark and fruit in serving bowls.
If necessary, sweeten the quark with honey.

Servings: 6

 Calories: 262

 Ready in 15 min

QUARK DESSERT

Ingredients:

2 cups low fat quark
1 tbsp honey liquid
1 tsp vanilla
1 cup kiwi fruit
3 tbsp pistachios
approx 10 mg purine

Instructions:

Add the quark, yogurt, honey, and vanilla powder to a bowl and mix well. Peel and slice Kiwi fruit, and roughly chop Pistachios.
Divide half of the quark into a bowl, place the kiwi slices on top, drizzle with the remaining quark, and top with the pistachio nuts.

Servings: 12

 Calories: 190

 Ready in 1h20min

VEGAN SWEET CHERRY BARS

Ingredients:

1 cup rye, spelled, or whole wheat flour
1 tsp powdered baking soda
1/2 tsp bicarbonate of soda
⅓ cup olive oil
¼ cup of cold water
2 tsp vanilla extract
1 cup sugar (cane or coconut)
Non-dairy milk, 1 1/4 cup
1 lemon's juice
1 ½ cup pitted and halved sweet cherries, fresh or frozen
approx 27 mg purine

Instructions:

Preheat the oven to 350 F / 170 C. A 9 x 13 rectangular baking dish should be lightly greased and lined on the bottom with a piece of rectangular parchment paper.

In a mixing bowl, combine the flours, baking powder and soda, and salt (or the bowl of a stand mixer).

In the bowl of a stand mixer or a big mixing bowl with an electric mixer, thoroughly combine the oil, water, sugar, and vanilla extract.

Mix in the non-dairy milk and lemon juice thoroughly. In two additions, add the dry ingredients, mixing on medium speed as you go. Pour 34% of the batter into your prepared baking dish until the batter is well mixed (no lumps visible).

Top with the halved frozen cherries. Drop the remaining batter on top of the cherries with a spoon. Coat cherries completely in batter, with a few peeking out from under them.

Place the baking dish in the oven. Bake for 45 minutes, or until golden brown on the edges, and put on top. Allow the cake to cool fully before serving.

Servings: 2

Calories: 445

Ready in 20 min

QUARK PANCAKES WITH FRUIT

Ingredients:

1 cup low-fat quark
3 eggs
4 tbsp spelled wholemeal flour
1 tsp vanilla extract
2 tbsp baking soda
1 tbsp of coconut oil
1 ½ cup of seasonal fruits
1 tbsp honey optional
approx 37 mg purine

Instructions:

Combine the quark and eggs in a mixing bowl, add the flour, vanilla, and baking soda, and stir until a dense dough forms.
In a non-stick pan, heat the oil, add 1 tbsp of batter to each pan, and bake 4 to 6 pancakes on both sides for 3–4 minutes over medium heat.
On the side, wash the fruit, cut it into small parts, and mix it well. Serve the pancakes with honey and fruit.

POTATOES AND VEGETABLES

Servings: 4

Calories: 254

Ready in 1 hour

POTATO GOULASH

Ingredients:

1 cup celeriac
1 red pepper,
1 yellow pepper
2 cups Waxy potatoes
2 onions, red
one garlic clove
1 tbsp of rapeseed oil
1 cup low sodium vegetable broth
1 tbsp powdered noble sweet paprika
cayenne
1 bunches of parsley
4 tbsp 3.5-percent-fat yogurt
approx 18 mg purine

Instructions:

Wash the peppers, split them in half, remove the seeds, and cut them into cubes. Celeriac and potatoes should be peeled and diced, and onions and garlic should be peeled and finely chopped. Heat the rapeseed oil for 4 minutes over medium heat, sauté the onions in a big saucepan. Fry for 3–4 minutes with the garlic, potatoes, and celery. With vegetable stock, deglaze the pan. Add the spices and cook the goulash for about 30 minutes, covered, over medium heat.

Cook for 5 minutes after adding the paprika to the potato goulash. Parsley should be washed, dried, and chopped roughly. Season the goulash with salt and pepper to taste, and serve with 1 tbsp yogurt and 1 tbsp parsley.

Servings: 4

 Calories: 123

 Ready in 1 hour

ROSEMARY-ROASTED POTATOES

Ingredients:

2 tbsp minced fresh rosemary
3 crushed garlic cloves
1 cup/package refrigerated red potato wedges (such as Simply Potatoes)
1 tbsp extra virgin olive oil
1/2 tsp powdered onion
A quarter tsp of salt
a quarter tsp of pepper
approx 22 mg purine

Instructions:

Preheat the oven to 250C / 500F.
Toss the potatoes with the remaining ingredients in a big mixing bowl.
Mix each potato wedge thoroughly to coat it in oil and seasonings.
Arrange the potato wedges on a foil-lined baking sheet.
Bake for 22 minutes, or until golden brown and soft. Serve immediately.

Serving: 6

Calories: 250

Ready in 1 hour

SWEET POTATO PONE

Ingredients:

1 cup white or orange fresh sweet potato peeled and grated
1 tsp ground cinnamon
1 tsp ground nutmeg
1 tsp vanilla essence
2 large eggs well beaten
2 tbsp fresh coconut grated or desiccated coconut
1 cup peeled pumpkin or squash grated
grated rind of half an orange
approx 36 mg purine

Instructions:

Grease and line an oblong tin 26cm x 18 cm x 4 cm with greaseproof paper. Preheat the oven to 190 C / 370 F. Combine all the ingredients in a large mixing bowl, and then stir in the eggs and set them aside.

Gently pour the mixture into the prepared tin. Bake for around 50-60 minutes. The finished cake should have an almost crunchy, golden topping with a firm base.

Servings: 2

 Calories: 390

 Ready in 1 hour 20 min

SCALLOPED POTATOES

Ingredients:

1 tbsp butter
2 cloves garlic
1 tbsp flour
1 cup milk
1 tsp salt
½ tsp pepper
3 Yukon potatoes, peeled
2 tbsps grated parmesan cheese
fresh parsley, chopped, for garnish
approx 38 mg purine

Instructions:

Preheat the oven to 350°F (180°C).
In a small pot, melt the butter and fry the garlic until it's just starting to brown.
Add the flour, salt, and pepper. Whisk until there are no lumps.
Slowly drizzle in the milk while constantly whisking to ensure a smooth mixture.
Bring to a boil, then remove from heat.
Slice the potatoes into about ⅛-inch (3 mm) thick slices, put them in a small baking dish.
Pour the sauce on top of the potatoes, then sprinkle with parmesan.
Bake for about 1 hour, until the top, is bubbly and golden brown.
Sprinkle chopped parsley on top, then serve.

Servings: 4

Calories: 471

Ready in 1 hour

KARTOFFEL-BLUMENKOHL-CURRY

Ingredients:

- 2 tbsp ginger
- 3 cups potatoes (7 potatoes)
- 1 chili pepper, orange
- two onions
- 2 tbsp ghee (clarified butter)
- 2 tsp turmeric powder (optional)
- 1 tsp cumin (black)
- 1 tsp coriander seeds, crushed
- ½ tsp mustard seed
- 2 cups vegetable broth
- cayenne pepper
- 5 tomatillos
- 1 mango (ripe)
- 2 tbsp parsley
- 2 whole curry leaves
- 1 tbsp coriander
- 1 tsp lemon juice
- Wholemeal flatbread 1 cup
- 1 cup plain yogurt (1.5 percent fat)
- 1 cup cauliflower
- approx 50 mg purine

Instructions:

Trim the cauliflower, wash it, and cut it into tiny florets. The potatoes should be peeled, washed, and cut into bits. Cook the cauliflower and potatoes in boiling water until soft. Rinse and set aside. Peel ginger and dice finely. Cut the chili half lengthwise, core it, wash it, and chop it. Onions should be peeled, halved, and cut into very fine strips. In a saucepan, melt the ghee. Three minutes over medium heat, sauté the onions with chili and ginger.

Saute for 2 minutes with turmeric, black cumin, coriander, and mustard seeds. Deglaze with stock. Add the cooked vegetables, season with salt and pepper, and cook, occasionally stirring, for about 10 minutes over low heat. Clean, wash, slice, and dice the tomatoes in the meantime. Dice the mango after peeling it and removing the pulp from the block. Wash and roughly chop the parsley, curry leaves, and coriander, reserving some for garnish; stir the remaining parsley, curry leaves, and coriander into the curry, along with the tomatoes and mango, and cook for another 15 minutes. Add lemon juice, salt, and pepper. Serve the curry with flatbread and yogurt, garnished with the set-aside herbs.

Servings: 4

Calories: 688

Ready 1 hour 15min

POTATO AND CHEESECAKE

Ingredients:

3 cups floury potatoes
2 tbsp fresh parsley
4 tbsp whole mountain cheese (low fat in dry matter)
2 cups mushrooms
4 shallots
3 tbsp spelled wholemeal flour
1 egg and 2 yolks of eggs
cayenne pepper
1 tsp spice nutmeg
2 tbsp breadcrumbs (whole grain)
rapeseed oil, 3 tbsp
½ cup of butter
1 tsp lemon juice
3 juniper berries, dried
approx 50 mg purine

Instructions:

Wash the potatoes and place them in a saucepan with enough water to cover them. Season with salt, bring to a boil, and boil for 25 minutes, covered, over medium heat. Meanwhile, wash the parsley, shake it dry, and chop it. Grate the cheese finely.
Clean the mushrooms and cut them in half or quarters, depending on how big they are. Shallots should be peeled, halved lengthwise, and cut into wedges. After draining and letting the water evaporate, peel and mash the potatoes. Combine the parsley, butter, flour, and egg in a mixing bowl. Season with salt, pepper, and freshly grated nutmeg, then mix until smooth. CONTINUE TO THE NEXT PAGE

Servings:

Calories:

Ready:

POTATO AND CHEESECAKE

Instructions:

Shape the mixture into 12–16 balls, flatten them, and roll them in breadcrumbs. In a pan, heat 12 tbsps of oil. 3–4 cakes should be fried in it for 3–4 minutes on each side over medium heat. Repeat the remaining mixture and keep the cakes warm in the oven at 80° C / 170 F.

Melt the butter in a saucepan over low heat, remove it, and set it aside to cool. Meanwhile, season the egg yolks with salt and pepper in a metal bowl with 1 tsp lemon juice.

In a saucepan, bring some water to a temperature of 80 degrees Celsius. Place the bowl containing the egg yolks on the saucepan and whisk the contents until creamy. While stirring, drizzle in the butter in a thin stream. Crush the juniper berries very finely in a mortar, then season the sauce with them. Cover and keep warm.

Brush the remaining oil on a grill pan and heat it. Grill the porcini mushrooms and shallots in it for 2-3 minutes over medium to high heat. Remove from the heat and season with salt and pepper to taste, as well as the remaining lemon juice. Serve the potato and cheese, as well as the mushroom mixture, on plates with the sauce.

Servings: 2

 Calories: 670

 Ready in 25 min

WINTER BOWL WITH POTATO

Ingredients:

1 tbsp rapeseed oil
½ tsp paprika powder
2 cups waxy potatoes
2 eggs
1 handful herbs (mixed)
1 cup fat-free quark
1 tbsp of linseed oil
cayenne
Lamb's lettuce
½ cup carrot,
1 tbsp hazelnut kernels
1 red onion, tiny
red wine vinegar, 2 tbsp
Vegetable broth, 2 tbsp
4 tbsp mustard
oil from hazelnuts
approx 58 mg purine

Instructions:

Boil the potatoes for 10 minutes. Then drain and set aside for 5 minutes to cool. After that, peel the potatoes and cut them into tiny cubes. In a pan, heat the rapeseed oil. Fry the potatoes for 5–7 minutes over medium heat, until crispy. Salt and paprika to taste, and keep warm in the pan.

Boil the eggs for 6–7 minutes in boiling water. Drain the eggs, rinse them in cold water, peel them, and break them lengthwise in half. Wash the herbs, shake them off, and cut them finely. Then combine quark, linseed oil, 3 tbsps water, salt, and pepper in a mixing bowl. The lamb's lettuce should be cleaned, washed, and dried.

Slice the carrot and wash it before cutting it into long strips. Chop the hazelnuts into small pieces. Peel the onion and finely chop it. Whisk together the vinegar, broth, butter, and mustard to make the dressing. After that, season with salt and pepper and add the onions. Combine the potatoes, carrots, lamb's lettuce, and eggs in two cups. Drizzle dressing over the salad and hazelnuts.

Servings: 4

Calories: 277

Ready 15 min

COTTAGE CHEESE ON POTATO TOAST

Ingredients:

2 sweet potatoes
1 carrot
3 basil stems
1 cup Cottage cheese (10 percent fat)
cayenne
powdered paprika
2 leaves red cabbage
approx 10 mg purine

Instructions:

Peel sweet potatoes, cut each into six thin slices, and toast for around 10 minutes in a toaster or bake for 10 minutes in a 200 C / 390 F preheated oven.

Clean, wash, and coarsely grate the carrot in the meantime. Wash the basil and shake it dry before plucking a few leaves aside and chopping the rest—season with salt, pepper, paprika, cottage cheese, carrot, and chopped basil.

Cut the red cabbage leaves into fine strips after washing them. Top sweet potato slices with cottage cheese and red cabbage strips, as well as basil leaves.

Servings: 4

Calories: 311

Ready 40 min

SWEET POTATO SALAD

Ingredients:

2 cups sweet potatoes (1 big sweet potato)
salt
Cheyenne pepper
1 tsp. curry powder
3 tbsp olive oil
1 cup spinach (baby)
1 lemon
2 tbsp walnut kernels
2 apples (green)
2 tbsp vegetable broth
4 tbsp quinoa puffed
1 handful chive herb
approx 36 mg purine

Instructions:

Peel and cut the sweet potato into bite-sized bits. Place on a baking sheet lined with baking paper and season with salt, pepper, one pinch of curry, and 1 tbsp of oil.

Bake the sweet potato for 20 minutes at 200°C /390 F in a preheated oven, turning it halfway through. Remove from the oven and set aside to cool for 10 minutes.

Meanwhile, clean and wash the spinach. Cut the lemon in half and squeeze the juice out. Chop the walnuts coarsely. Apples should be cleaned, washed, quartered, and cored before being cut into small pieces and drizzled with half the lemon juice.

Combine the remaining lemon juice, salt, pepper, and the remaining oil to make a dressing.

Combine the prepared ingredients with the dressing in a mixing bowl and divide them into four bowls. Sprinkle Quinoa and chive over the salad.

Servings: 4

Calories: 505

Ready 1 hour

SAUERKRAUT KUMPIR

Ingredients:

8 big waxy potatoes
2 tsp rapeseed oil
2 cups sauerkraut
1 cup plain yogurt (1.5 percent fat)
1 tsp caraway seed
salt
cayenne pepper
2 carrots
1 pear
1 tbsp of lemon juice
4 coriander stems
2 tbsp walnut kernels
One piece of 50 g gouda (45 percent fat in dry matter)
4 tbsp butter (room temperature)
approx 38 mg purine

Instructions:

Wash the potatoes, poke them several times with a fork, brush with oil, and bake for 45 minutes at 200 C / 390 F in a preheated oven until tender. Meanwhile, remove the sauerkraut and combine it with the yogurt and caraway seeds, seasoning to taste. Clean, wash, and grate the carrots and pears coarsely, then combine with the lemon juice. Wash the coriander, shake it out, and chop the leaves.
Roughly chop walnuts and roast for 3 minutes in a hot pan without fat over medium heat. Remove the potatoes from the oven, cut them lengthwise, and use a fork to loosen the insides. Combine butter and Gouda cheese in a mixing bowl. Fill the potatoes with sauerkraut, pear, carrot mixture, and roasted walnuts and coriander before serving.

Servings: 5 | Calories: 420 | Ready 40 min

FRIED POTATO AND ASPARAGUS PAN

Ingredients:
2 cups green asparagus
5 shallots
3 cups small waxy potatoes
1 tbsp clarified butter
3 parsley stems
cayenne pepper
approx 18 mg purine

Instructions:
Wash potatoes and boil for 15 minutes in salted water.
Meanwhile, wash the asparagus, peel the bottom third, and trim the woody ends. Boil the asparagus for 8 minutes in salted boiling water. Drain, and break into pieces diagonally.
Drain the potatoes, let them cool down before cutting them half lengthwise.
Cut shallots into wedges after peeling them.
In a high pan, melt the clarified butter. Fry the potatoes over medium heat, frequently turning, for 10 minutes, or until golden brown.
Wash the parsley, shake it dry and chop it. Combine the shallots and potatoes in a pan and cook for 4 minutes. Stir in the asparagus and cook for another 2 minutes, turning frequently.
Add salt, pepper, and parsley to the fried potato and asparagus pan.

Servings: 6 Calories: 460 Ready 1,20 hour

SWEET POTATO AND CARROT GRATIN

Ingredients:
1 cup milk
2 cups sweet potatoes
1 ½ cup carrots
½ cup creme fraiche low fat
3 eggs
half bunch fresh thyme
½ cup Gruyère cheese (1 piece)
freshly ground pepper
nutmeg, freshly grated
2 tbsp pumpkin seeds
approx 23 mg purine

Instructions:
Peel and thinly slice the sweet potatoes and carrots. In a baking dish, alternately layer the vegetable slices.
Combine the milk, crème fraîche, and eggs in a large mixing bowl. Pick the leaves off the thyme after it has been washed and dried.
To taste, combine half of the thyme and half of the cheese in a mixing bowl: salt, pepper, and nutmeg.
Pour the egg milk over the vegetables and mix well. On top, sprinkle the remaining cheese and pumpkin seeds. Beak for 45 minutes at 180 C/350 F in a preheated oven. Serve with the remaining thyme as a garnish.

Servings: 4

 Calories: 475

 Ready 45 min

PEANUT AND SWEET POTATO SOUP

Ingredients:

3 cups sweet potatoes
1 cup carrots
1 shallot
2 cloves garlic
1 red chili pepper
2 tbsp olive oil
1 tsp turmeric powder (optional)
1 tsp curry powder
2 cups vegetable broth, cayenne
2 cups coconut beverage
1 cup pak choi baby
4 tbsp peanut kernels, roasted
2 tbsp fresh parsley
2 tbsp Peanut butter
2 tbsp 3.5-percent-fat yogurt
1 tbsp black sesame seeds
approx 42 mg purine

Instructions:

Prepare the sweet potatoes and carrots by peeling, washing, and dicing them. Shallots and garlic should be peeled and diced finely. Cut the chili half lengthwise, core it, wash it, and chop it.

In a saucepan, heat the oil. In it, sauté shallot, garlic, and chili for a few minutes. Cook for 3 minutes on medium heat. Sauté sweet potatoes and carrots for 4 minutes, seasoning with turmeric and curry powder. Then add broth to deglaze, season with salt and pepper, and top with a coconut drink. Cook the soup for 20 minutes over low heat.

Meanwhile, clean and wash the pak choy before cutting it into strips. Chop the peanuts into small pieces. Parsley should be washed, dried, and chopped. Cook for 5–8 minutes after adding the pakchoi and peanut butter to the soup. Season with salt and pepper.

Drizzle 1 tsp yogurt over the soup and garnish with the remaining peanuts, sesame seeds, and parsley on deep plates.

Servings: 4   Calories: 241   Ready 30 min

POTATO AND RADISH SALAD

Ingredients:

1 cup vegetable broth
4 cups waxy potatoes
1 mild onion
4 tbsp apple cider vinegar
1 tbsp of grainy mustard
cayenne
1 cup radish
2 handfuls of Rocket
half bunch chives
rapeseed oil, 3 tbsp
approx 24 mg purine

Instructions:

Boil the potatoes for 20–30 minutes. Then drain, let them cool, peel and slice.
Peel and finely dice the onion. Bring the broth to a boil, then add in the onion. Remove from heat and set aside for 5 minutes to steep. Season the marinade with salt and pepper after adding the vinegar and mustard. Prepare the radishes by washing, cleaning, and slicing them. The Rocket should be washed and cleaned before being shaken dry. Break the chives into rolls after washing them. Combine the marinade with potatoes and set aside
for 30 minutes to steep.
Mix all ingredients in a salad bowl, season to taste, and serve.

Servings: 4

 Calories: 80

 Ready 35 min

AUBERGINES

Ingredients:

2 large aubergines
½ medium onion chopped
2 cloves garlic minced
2 medium tomatoes chopped
1 tsp curry powder
freshly ground black pepper
small bunch coriander finely chopped
approx 20 mg purine

Instructions:

Wash aubergines and make slits in them with a knife, then stuff the slits with the garlic and roast over a gas hob or grill until soft.
Slice in half, scrape out the pulp, and mash with all the ingredients using a fork.
Gently cook in a non-stick frying pan for 5 -7 minutes. Serve in a roti or as a side dish to curried meat or fish.

www.ingramcontent.com/pod-product-compliance
Lightning Source LLC
Chambersburg PA
CBHW081354080526
44588CB00016B/2494